I0434998

Health Benefits of Rye

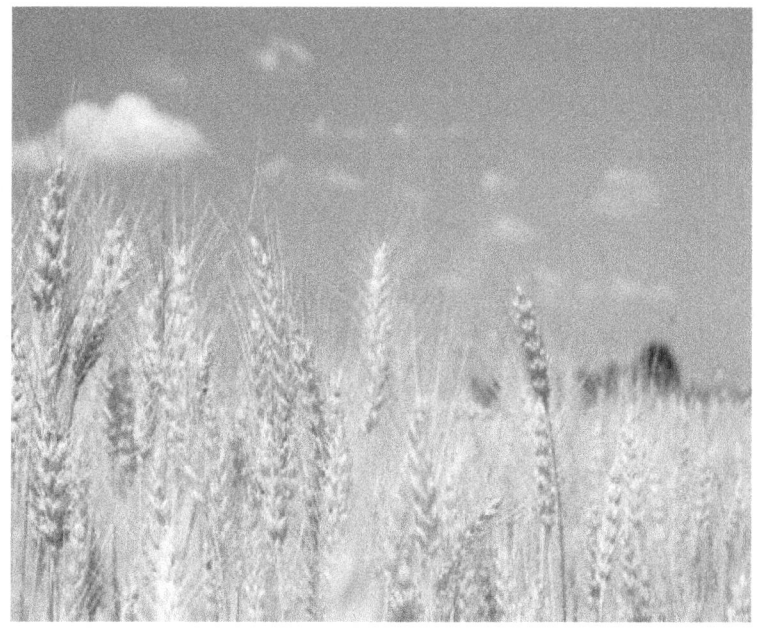

Healthy Living Series

M. Usman

Mendon Cottage Books

JD-Biz Publishing

All Rights Reserved.

No part of this publication may be reproduced in any form or by any means, including scanning, photocopying, or otherwise without prior written permission from JD-Biz Corp Copyright © 2014

All Images Licensed by Fotolia and 123RF.

Disclaimer

The information is this book is provided for informational purposes only. It is not intended to be used and medical advice or a substitute for proper medical treatment by a qualified health care provider. The information is believed to be accurate as presented based on research by the author.

The contents have not been evaluated by the U.S. Food and Drug Administration or any other Government or Health Organization and the contents in this book are not to be used to treat cure or prevent disease.

The author or publisher is not responsible for the use or safety of any diet, procedure or treatment mentioned in this book. The author or publisher is not responsible for errors or omissions that may exist.

Warning

The Book is for informational purposes only and before taking on any diet, treatment or medical procedure, it is recommended to consult with your primary health care provider.

Check out some of the other Healthy Gardening Series books at Amazon.com

Gardening Series on Amazon

Check out some of the other Health Learning Series books at Amazon.com

Health Learning Series on Amazon

Table of Contents

Preface.. 4

Getting Started 5

Chapter # 1: Intro 5

Chapter # 2: Nutritional Worth 8

Chapter # 3: Varieties of Rye.................................... 11

Chapter # 4: Selection & Storage.............................. 14

Health Benefits.. 16

Chapter # 1: Lowers Type-2 Diabetes Risk 16

Chapter # 2: Prevents Gallstones 19

Chapter # 3: Cardiovascular Protection 21

Chapter # 4: Lowers Cancer Risk 24

Recipes 26

Chapter # 1: Homemade Rye Bread........................... 26

Chapter # 2: Herb & Walnut Rolls............................ 28

Chapter # 3: Rye Rounds 30

Conclusion 31

References.. 32

Preface

While most other cereal grains can be traced back to prehistoric cultures, rye is a crop that has caught the attention of the world, not that long ago. In recorded history, rye was first grown in Germany, back in 400BC; this is not that long ago, considering wheat was being grown in Jordan as far back as 7500 BC! Rye is believed to have been originated from a class of Asian wild grass found in Iran, Armenia and Syria. The Roman philosopher and author, Pliny the Elder stated that rye was a food that wasn't consumed until every other food item had been exhausted. Despite its ruggedness, rye slowly started gaining importance in Scandinavian and Eastern European cultures, and now, science has discovered that rye is a very nutritious cereal that can keep the body fit. More and more people are getting excited about this crop and are now looking for ways to incorporate it into their diet.

This book comprehensively explains every aspect of rye & how it benefits the body.

Getting Started

Chapter # 1: Intro

Rye is a cereal grain with a strong, unique flavor and visual characteristics similar to that of wheat, but with more length & slimness; the color of the cereal varies from yellow-brown to green to gray. Like many other cereals, rye also comes in many forms, like:

- Whole rye berry

- Rye flour

- Rye flakes

- Fermented rye products

These have been explained in detail in the coming chapters. In comparison to wheat, rye is often considered healthier as it is much more difficult to separate the bran & germ from the rye grain, implying that the cereal will pack more nutrients in flour form. The bran of a grain is the multi-layered outer skin of the edible part of the grain known as the kernel. The bran may seem undesirable to consume but it must be known that it is filled with plenty of vital anti-oxidants, fibers and B-vitamins. Same is the case with the germ that is the embryo of the grain, having the ability to sprout into a new plant; the germ is packed with B-vitamins, minerals, proteins and healthy fats. Furthermore, rye bread is also much denser than wheat bread due to less elastic gluten, meaning less gas will be held during the leavening process.

As it was said earlier, throughout history, rye has been considered a second class food and therefore has been mostly used to feed livestock. Even though this trend is changing, especially in European countries, still much of the rye grown in USA is used to feed animals. The majority of the world's rye comes from Poland, China, Russia, Denmark and Canada.

Overviews of mineral-specific benefits have been given in the next section, however, a very exciting benefit of rye must be discussed here. Rye has the ability to encourage the production of a substance necessary for a healthy colon, butyric acid. Studies have shown that this particular acid helps keep the intestinal linings healthy and up to the mark, therefore, relieving symptoms of ailments like Crohn's disease, inflammatory bowel disease, etc. Now for the more interesting part; studies have also shown that the acid has the ability to turn cancerous cells into normal cells. This is quite a unique feature as most substances either cause the cancer cell to kill itself or kill the cancer cells themselves, but butyric acid seems to save the cell from destruction by normalizing its function and returning it back to its previous state.

Other benefits of rye include:

- Lowering the risk of cardiovascular diseases like heart failure.

- Lowering cholesterol levels and optimizing heart health by controlling blood pressure.

- An extremely healthy class of compounds in rye i.e. lignans work to lower the risk of certain cancers. They are highly effective in reducing mammary tumors and slowing the growth of cancerous cells in the breast and colon. Also, by improving the bowel function rye reduces the risk of colorectal cancer.

- Lignans also act as antioxidants and help in reducing the occurrence of vaginal dryness and hot flashes in postmenopausal women.

- Rye helps in inhibiting the initiation of coronary artery complications as well as osteoporosis.

- Rye bread improves fecal output in both men and women.

- Rye provides a feeling of fullness to the consumer and satiety for much longer durations, helping those on diets and indirectly aiding to weight loss.

- It also helps trigger a quick insulin response, making it an efficient alternate for diabetics.

- Many other diseases include sclerosis, adenitis, abscess, vascular diseases, tonsillitis, constipation, enteritis, and contusion are also dealt with inclusion of rye into everyday diet.

The next chapter provides a nutrient-specific benefit overview so it will make more sense as to why rye helps the body.

Chapter # 2: Nutritional Worth

Rye is very good in providing the body with dietary fiber, minerals like phosphorous & magnesium, and B-vitamins. A great feature of rye is its 4 to 1 ratio magnesium to calcium content. This is an important quality as many Americans nowadays focus only on their calcium intake, but are quite ignorant when it comes to magnesium. If this ratio is upset, it can lead to many problems for the body like kidney stones, calcification of arteries that can lead to arteriosclerosis, and the calcification of joints that can cause arthritis. Magnesium, a heart-friendly mineral, helps normalizes the ratio and brings back balance to the body.

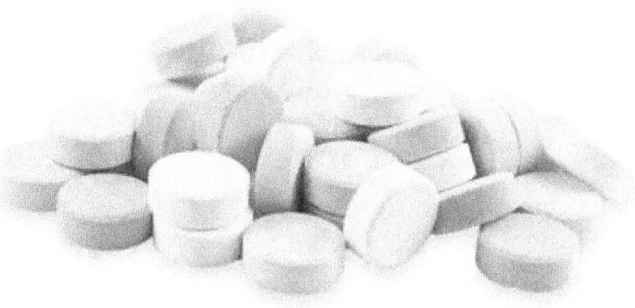

Rye, being high in fiber, is a great food for diabetics as the high fiber content decreases the frequency of spikes in blood sugar level. Rye also helps in minimizing the symptoms of irritable bowels syndrome through its high fiber content. Studies have also shown that fiber can reduce the risk of colon cancer. The fiber adds bulk to the stool that causes the toxins in the body to excrete more rapidly. If the stool remains in the body for too long, the toxins are reabsorbed by the body causing inflammations that eventually become a factor in the development of colon cancer. The fiber therefore, not only prevents colon cancer from developing but also causes the inflammation in the digestive tract to cease.

A detailed account of the nutritional wellness of rye is given in the following table. The amount taken is 1 cup or 169 grams. The table also includes the percent daily values that are for adults or children over the age of 3.

Calorie Information		
Nutrient	**Amount**	**% DV**
Total Calories	566 (2370 kJ)	
From Carbohydrates	455 (1905 kJ)	28%
From Fat	35.4 (148 kJ)	
From Proteins	76.1 (319 kJ)	
Carbohydrates		
Nutrient	**Amount**	**% DV**
Total Carbohydrates	118 g	39%
Dietary Fiber	24.7 g	99%
Starch	0.0 g	
Sugar	1.8 g	
Fats & Fatty Acids		
Nutrient	**Amount**	**% DV**
Total Fat	4.2 g	7%
Saturated Fat	0.5 g	2%
Mono-saturated Fat	0.5 g	
Polyunsaturated Fat	1.9 g	
Total Omega-3 Fatty acids	265 mg	
Total Omega-6 Fatty acids	1619 mg	
Proteins		
Nutrient	**Amount**	**% DV**
Protein	24.9 g	50%
Vitamins		
Nutrient	**Amount**	**% DV**
Vitamin A	18.6 IU	0%
Vitamin C	0.0 mg	0%
Vitamin E	2.2 mg	11%

Vitamin K	10.0 mcg	12%
Thiamin	0.5 mg	36%
Riboflavin	0.4 mg	25%
Niacin	7.2 mg	36%
Vitamin B6	0.5 mg	25%
Folate	101 mcg	25%
Vitamin B12	0.0 mg	0%
Pantothenic Acid	2.5 mg	25%
Choline	51.4 mg	

Minerals		
Nutrient	**Amount**	**% DV**
Calcium	55.8 mg	6%
Iron	4.5 mg	25%
Magnesium	204 mg	51%
Phosphorus	632 mg	63%
Potassium	446 mg	13%
Sodium	10.1 mg	0%
Zinc	6.3 mg	42%
Copper	0.8 mg	38%
Manganese	4.5 mg	226%
Selenium	59.7 mcg	85%

Chapter # 3: Varieties of Rye

In the Northern Hemisphere, most rye is "winter rye", meaning it is planted in the months of autumn, begins development during springtime, and gets harvested by August. Same as other grains, rye also comes in many forms; however there are many kinds of rye products that can some time become confusing.

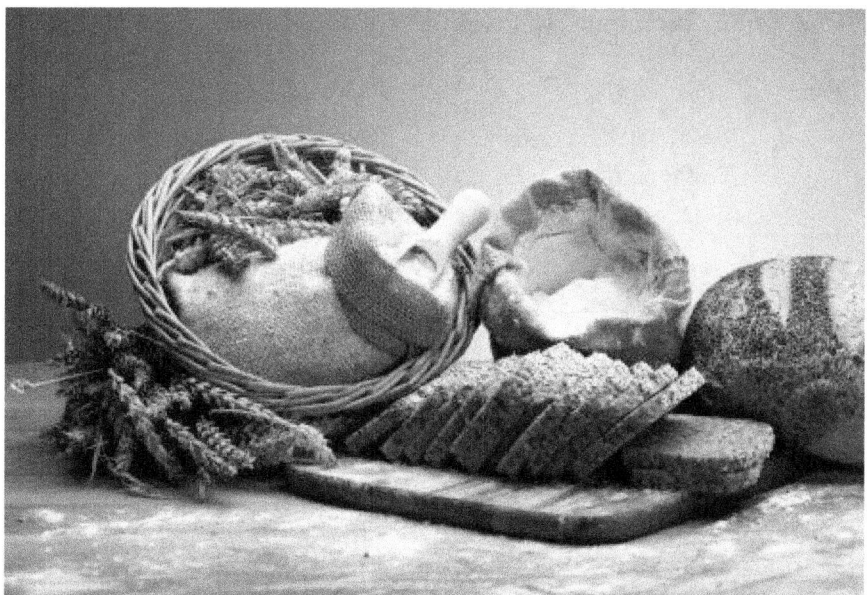

- **Rye Berries:**

    Whole kernels or the edible part of the grain is referred to as "rye berries". When rye comes straight from the field, it has an inedible hull which must be removed before rye can be eaten or even milled. In rye, the starchy endosperm makes up about 83% of the whole kernel, the germ makes up 2-3% while the outer bran constitutes about 10-15%.

- **Cracked Rye/Rye chops:**

    Ever heard of steel cut oats or cracked wheat? Well rye chops are the rye equivalent of these products. The whole kernel or the rye berry is cracked into a few pieces; this is done as the new form is easier to cook as compared to an intact rye berry.

- **Rye Flakes:**

Rye flakes are produced just like rolled oats; rye berries are steamed, rolled and then finally dried. Rye flakes can be cooked into porridge, added into baked goods or used just like rolled oats.

Now, the different types of rye flours and rye meals:

i. **White rye flour:**

Rye flour that consists only of the endosperm is known as white rye flour. Just like refined wheat flour, rye flour also lacks many of the original nutrients found in the kernel.

ii. **Light rye flour or cream:**

Inclusion of small traces of bran in white rye flour makes it into light rye flour or cream.

iii. **Medium rye flour:**

If more bran is included in the white rye flour, medium rye flour is obtained which has many of the original characteristics of the rye.

iv. **Dark rye flour:**

Dark rye is sometimes also referred to as whole grain flour; this term varies from miller to miller. Some make it 100% whole flour while others include just some of the layers of the endosperm and a little bran. For some, dark rye is just a mixture of the leftovers from light, white and medium rye flour.

v. **Rye meal:**

This is the best term for whole grain rye flour. Rye meal contains the bran, endosperm and germ of the original rye berry; it can be ground to fine, medium or coarse levels.

vi. **Pumpernickel:**

Coarse, whole grain rye flour is known as pumpernickel. It is also the name of the traditional German bread.

Chapter # 4: Selection & Storage

Rye flour can be found in the natural food section of many large grocery store chains; a greater variety of rye products however are mostly found at health or natural food grocers. Whole or cracked rye berries are usually found in bulk bins and small one pound bags. When buying any cereal from a bulk bin, make sure that it is covered, kept in a cool & dry place and the store has a high turnover rate, otherwise you would be buying stale rye.

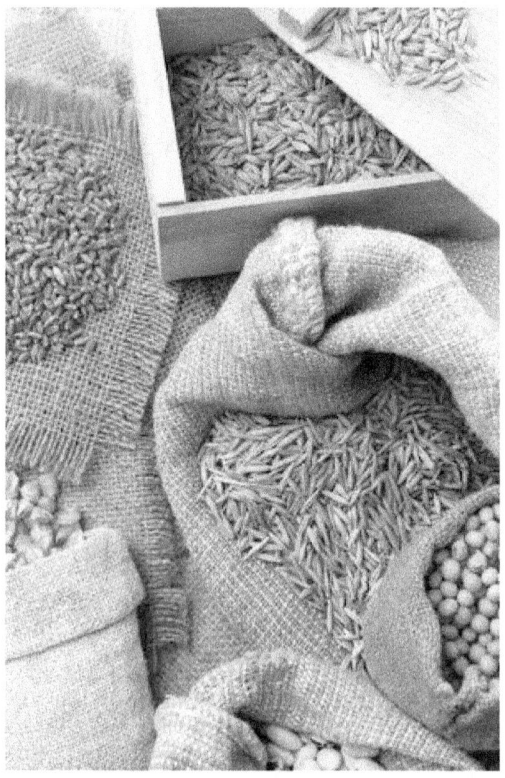

After buying the flour it can be kept well in a sealed container that is stored in a cool, dark and moisture-free place. The original paper package is fine for long term storage as long as the packet has not been opened. After that, any moisture can seriously damage the grain and decrease its shelf life. Here are a few ways to increase the shelf life of rye:

- After the packaging has been opened, rye flour must be stored in a sealed container that must be kept in a cool and dry cabinet.

- The refrigerator is an excellent storage area for rye flour but the use of sealed containers is equally important to prevent the flour from absorbing moisture along with odors and flavors from other food.

- If long-term storage is what you desire, then the freezer is the best location for that. Use sealed plastic containers or freezer bags to preserve freshness.

If stored properly, white rye flour can last longer than the whole one but with that said, flour that smells or does not look good must not be used as it would cause more harm and would taste awful.

When dealing with rye berries, make sure to rinse and wash them so they have no dirt. Rye berries are best cooked using 1 part rye with three to four parts of boiling water. Once the water reaches its boiling point, lower the heat, cover the container and let the rye simmer for an hour.

Rye bread is also widely available at bakeries. It is made up with either light or dark rye flours. Light rye flour bread tends to have a tan color, a light flavor and contains only a small amount of outer bran. Dark rye bread however, has a deeper color, intense flavor and is made of all of the outer bran of the kernel.

Health Benefits

Chapter # 1: Lowers Type-2 Diabetes Risk

Diabetes is described as a group of metabolic diseases that are highlighted by high blood sugar that could be a result of either inadequate production of blood sugar or improper response by the body's cells to insulin, or in some cases both. Diabetes is often accompanied by frequent urination, and increased thirst & hunger.

There are three types of diabetes:

Type-1 Diabetes – The body is unable to produce enough insulin.

Type-2 Diabetes – The body does not produce enough insulin for normal function or the cells do not respond to this production. This is the most common of all three.

Gestational Diabetes – Some women have very high levels of glucose in their blood and their bodies do not have the right amount of insulin to transport this glucose into their cells resulting in diabetes; it is most common during pregnancy.

Where does rye come in all this?

Rye is a rich source of the mineral magnesium that acts as a helper to many reactions in the body, including those that involve the use of glucose or insulin. Regular consumption of whole grains can reduce the risk of type-2 diabetes, according to a research published in *Diabetes Care*. In the 8 year trial that involved 41,186 participants; the Black Women's Health Study's research data showed clear inverse relations between calcium, magnesium and other food items' relation to type-2 diabetes. The risk of type-2 diabetes was 31% lower in women who ate whole grains more frequently than women eating the least amount of whole grains. It was also found that foods rich in magnesium other than whole foods had a lower effect on the reduction of the risk of type-2 diabetes.

A study published in the September 2009 issue of *Nutrition Journal* confirmed the working of whole grain rye in treatment of diabetes. The study aimed to explore the mechanism by which rye products induced a reduced post-prandial insulin response that lead to improvement in the condition of diabetics. 12 healthy subjects were chosen for this study and each was given a flour based product made from rye's endosperm, whole grain or bran.

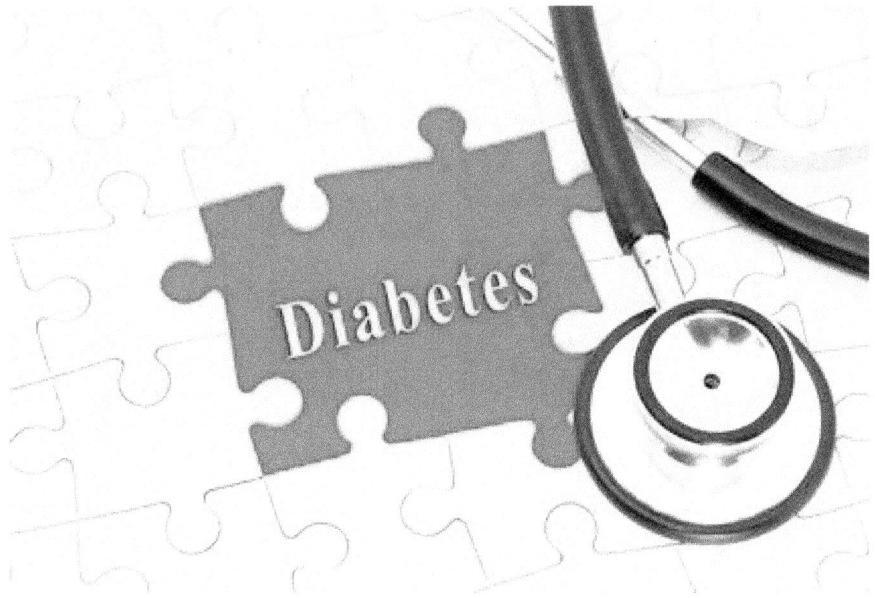

The product was produced using different methods: simulated sour-dough baking and boiling or baking; they were served as breakfasts in a randomized order governed by a cross-over design. The reference for the study was a meal of white wheat bread. Different substances in the blood like glucose, insulin and plasma ghrelin were measured during 180 minutes. For a more organized analysis the Glycemic profile was used; the higher the score, the longer the energy provided by the food lasts in the body. The results showed that the endosperm and whole grain rye products were able to improve the Glycemic profile and induce a low acute insulinaemic response in participants. This means that rye products have appetite & blood sugar regulating properties that are not only beneficial for a normal person but also for a diabetic.

Another study illustrated the effect of grains including rye on inflammation markers that are believed to have a negative effect on glucose & insulin levels, which can increase the risk of type-2 diabetes. Researchers from the University of Kuopio in Finland carried out trials on 47 adults with metabolic syndrome by dividing them in to two groups. One group was given a diet of oats, white bread, and potato, while the other rye bread and pasta for a period of 12 weeks. Glucose and insulin levels in the two groups were determined in 19 individuals in the first run. Blood samples of the participants were taken both before and after the 12 week period; the results showed that participants of the rye group had lower insulin, GIP and C-peptide responses compared to the oat group. In simple words, there was a decrease in inflammation in the rye group that showed that it had potential to reduce the risk of type-2 diabetes in sufferers of metabolic syndrome.

Chapter # 2: Prevents Gallstones

When substances in the gallbladder or bile duct accumulate for a certain period of time, they form lumps or stones known as gallstones. Chemicals in the gallbladder like calcium, cholesterol, calcium carbonate and bilirubinate solidify into either several small stones or a large stone. Researchers have described this situation as trying to squeeze a golf ball through a straw! There are two types of gallstones:

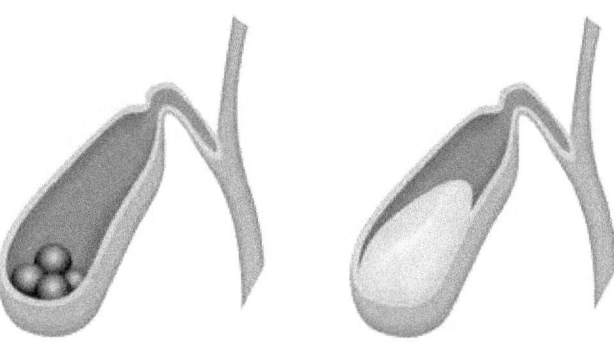

i. **Cholesterol gallstones** – formed by too much accumulation of cholesterol

ii. **Pigment gallstones** – formed when the bilirubin content in the bile increases to unacceptable levels.

Eating foods high in insoluble fiber can help cure this problem. A study dedicated to this research was published in the *American Journal of Gastroenterology*. The study was designed to analyze the overall intake of fiber along with the types of fiber consumed over a 16 year period in about 69,000 women; the *Nurses' Health Study* was used as a medium for data collection. In a nutshell, it was found that women who consumed the most fiber throughout this time period (both types) had a 13% lower risk of developing gallstones. When it came to those who consumed more insoluble fiber, it was found that chances of curing gallstones increased by 17%. Furthermore, it was concluded that the protection offered by grains was proportional to the dose; a 5 gram increase in the fiber intake dropped the risk by 10%. The insoluble fiber not only speeded the intestinal tract's transit time period but also reduced the secretion of toxic bile acids that lead to the formation of gallstones, increased insulin sensitivity, and lowered triglycerides. Rye being high in insoluble fiber content can therefore help people with the risk of developing gallstones.

Chapter # 3: Cardiovascular Protection

The cardiovascular system is a sophisticated network of organs and blood vessels responsible for transporting nutrients and removing gaseous waste materials from the body. The system is composed of the heart, the blood vessels and blood. The cardiovascular system is a necessity for life and if any part of the system becomes damaged, there is an immediate threat to the mortality of the person.

One of the most vital benefits of rye is that it lowers high cholesterol levels. It does so by binding to toxins in the colon and removing them from the body. When fiber binds to bile salts in the intestinal tract and removes them, the body starts to make more of these salts, which is good. In order to produce these salts, a breakdown of cholesterol is required. It is by this mechanism, that rye achieves lower cholesterol levels.

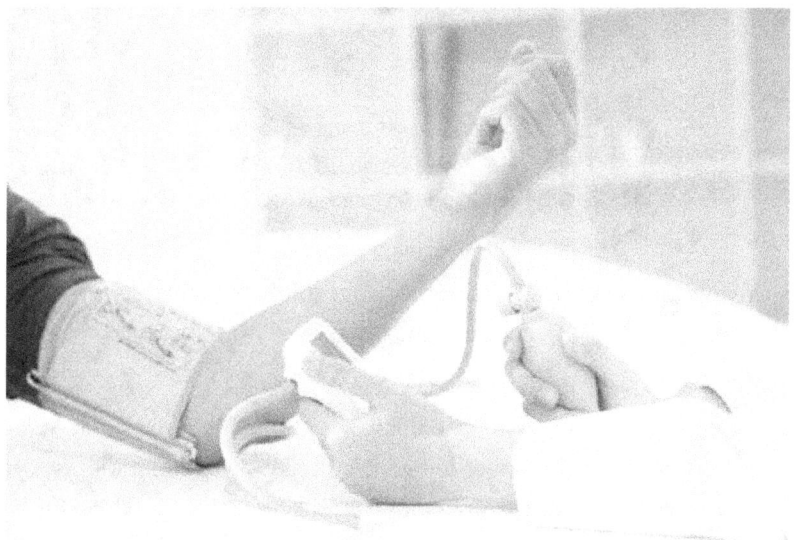

Heart failure is a cardiovascular risk that has become the leading cause of hospitalization among the elder population of the United States. Success through drug treatments has shown partial benefits and there is no confirmation as to whether Statin drugs are safe for the patient or not. A follow up of the discharged patients has showed that 37.3% of the discharged patients died during the first year while the rest died during the next five years. The consumption of whole grains like rye has had a positive effect on reducing the risk of high blood pressure and heart attack. This prompted the researchers at Harvard to look into the effects of cereal consumption and heart failure risk. The study was carried out with the help of Physicians Health Study for a period of 19.6 years and on 21,736 participants. Factors such as age, lifestyle, and consumption of vitamins, exercise and medical history were accounted for and it was found that men who incorporated a bowl of cereal like rye flakes in their morning diet had a 29% lower risk of heart failure then those who consumed the least amount of cereals.

There were also significant benefits for postmenopausal women with high blood pressure, cholesterol, and other signs of CVD. A 3 year study of over 200 postmenopausal women was published in the American Heart Journal; it showed that women who ate at least 6 servings of whole grains like rye in a week experienced:

i.   Slowed progress in the development of the disease atherosclerosis, the buildup of plaque in blood vessels that causes reduced blood flow.

ii.   And less progression in stenosis, which is narrowing of the arterial passageways.

It was also found that the whole grains were solely responsible for this effect and the intake of fruits, vegetables and grains had no effect on the reduction of CVD risk.

For decades it was believed by scientists that ultimately, genes determined a person's destiny; if you've inherited genes that give you heart disease, you will at some point of your life develop heart disease. But more recently it has been found that genes can be toggled on or off. The current research has shown that your lifestyle and diet alone can help in keeping the switch off by "down-regulating" genes. Scientists at University of Kuopio studied the effects of oat/potato/wheat diet compared to a pasta/rye diet for 12 weeks in 47 individuals. After the 12 week time period it was discovered that the rye/pasta group down-regulated 71 genes, including those linked with apoptosis that is programmed cell death and insulin signaling. In comparison, the other group down-regulated 62 genes related to stress, interleukin pathway and cytokine-chemokine-mediated immunity. Also there was an improvement in the insulinogenic index after consumption of the rye/pasta diet whereas body weight was unchanged in both groups.

Rye also contains protective phytonutrients lignans that are converted to mammalian lignans through friendly flora in the body. One of the products of this flora is enterolactone that is believed to have benefits like protection against breast cancer and heart disease. When blood levels of 800 postmenopausal women were checked for enterolactone, the women who ate the most amounts of whole grains, like rye, carried the greatest amount of the protective lignans in them.

Chapter # 4: Lowers Cancer Risk

Cancer is a disease characterized by uncontrolled growth of abnormal cells in different parts of the body. The abnormal cells spread throughout the body using the blood and lymph systems. There are over 100 different types of cancer and most of them are named after the organ in which they originate.

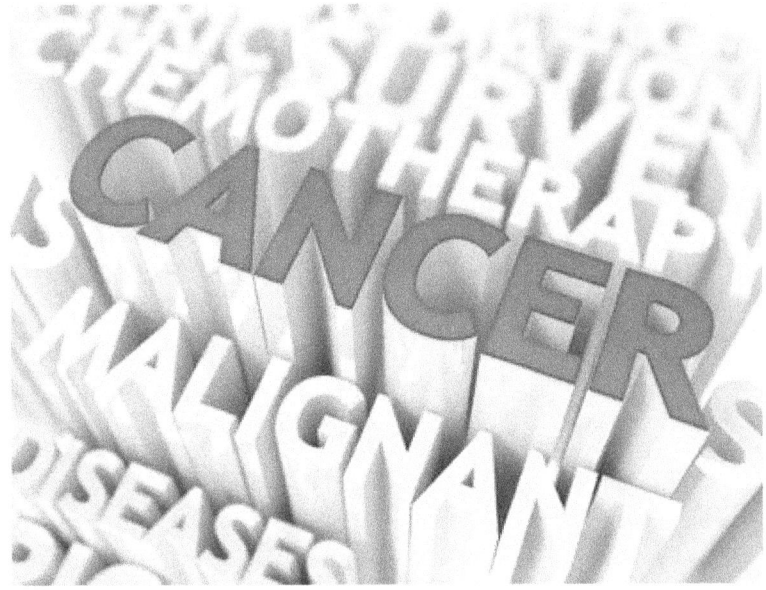

The American Institute for Cancer Research holds an International Conference on food, nutrition and cancer. In one such conference, Rui Hai Liu, M.D, PhD and his colleagues from the Cornell University, showed that whole grains had many health-promoting substances known as phytonutrients that have been overlooked by scientists. For years, researchers have only focused on the antioxidant power of phytonutrients that are "free" in form. These "free" phytonutrients dissolve quickly and are immediately absorbed into the blood whereas the "bound" form remains attached to the walls of the plant cells and are absorbed into the blood stream with the help of intestinal bacteria during digestion. Phenolics were another class of antioxidants that have the ability to prevent multiple diseases. When Dr. Liu and his colleagues measured the amount of phenolics and their presence in bound or free form in fruits and vegetables, it was found that the 76% of the total phenolics found were in free form. In comparison, free phenolics in whole grains accounted for less than 1% while the remaining phenolics were in bound form. This showed that the ability of whole grains to act as antioxidants had been severely underestimated and there were many more benefits of rye that can still be reaped. The team's findings explained the reason as to why populations who consume more whole grains have less risk of colorectal cancer. Antioxidant activity of these chemicals helps take care of harmful free radicals in the body that can cause damage to cells that eventually lead to cancer. The phytochemicals in whole grains like rye act in synergistic manner and ward off diseases that can lead to development of tumors.

Another situation in which rye is extremely effective is menopause. Rye packs up a lignan that has phytoestrogenic properties. In the body, phytoestrogens act like natural compounds entrusted with the task of normalizing estrogen activity. Even though the effects of phytoestrogens is much weaker than the natural variant, it is still enough to help prevent breast cancer. Some women have reported reduction in uncomfortable symptoms caused by plummeting estrogen levels like hot flashes. On the other hand, too much estrogen is also dangerous for the body and can lead to breast cancer; in this situation rye's lignans step up, and block out the more powerful estrogens and with that, bring down the risk of breast cancer in postmenopausal women.

Researchers analyzed the UK Women's Cohort study and found out that of the 35,972 participants, those who ate a fiber rich diet like rye had a significant protection against breast cancer. Pre-menopausal women, who consumed more than 30 grams of fiber a day, halved their risk of getting breast cancer compared to those consuming less than 20 grams a day. Fiber from whole grains like rye was most effective as consumption of less than 13 grams of whole grain fiber resulted in a 41% reduction in the risk of development of breast cancer.

Recipes

Chapter # 1: Homemade Rye Bread

Makes: 10 to 12 servings

Prep time: 30 minutes

Cooking time: 45 minutes

Inactive for: 2 hours

Ingredients:

- 1 envelope dry yeast
- 1 tablespoon sugar
- 1 egg
- 1 large egg, beaten
- 3 tablespoons melted butter
- 1 cup warm milk
- *1 cup rye flour*
- 1 ½ teaspoons salt
- 1 tablespoon caraway seeds
- 2 ½ cups bleached all-purpose flour
- 1 teaspoon vegetable oil

Directions:

First, combine the sugar, yeast, egg, melted butter, and milk in an electric mixer bowl with a dough hook fitted. Beat on low speed for about a minute and add salt, all-purpose flour, caraway seeds, and rye flour afterwards. Beat again for a minute, until the flour becomes incorporated. Then, beat the mixture at a medium speed so that it forms a bowl and climbs up the dough hook. Remove the dough from the bowl and make it into a smooth ball using your hands. Place the dough into a lightly oiled bowl and move it so it becomes covered with oil at all sides. Cover with a plastic wrap and set aside in a warm place until the size doubles (1 hour). Preheat the oven to 350 degrees Fahrenheit and grease a 5 ½ x 9 inches baking pan. Remove the dough and place it onto a lightly floured surface. Knead the dough several times if necessary. Place the dough into the baking pan and cover it with a plastic wrap; set aside in a draft-free place until the size doubles and then use a pastry brush to brush an egg over the top of the dough. Bake for 45 minutes and cool on a rack.

Chapter # 2: Herb & Walnut Rolls

Makes: 8 rolls

Prep time: 30 minutes

Cooking time: 10 – 30 minutes

Ingredients:

- 300 g brown bread flour
- 200 g spelt flour
- *50 g rye flour*
- 50 g white bread flour
- 1 ½ teaspoon salt
- 1 tablespoon chopped fresh thyme
- 1 tablespoon chopped fresh sage
- 2 tablespoon chopped fresh parsley
- 1 tablespoon chopped fresh rosemary
- 2 sachets dried yeast (fast acting)
- 2 tablespoons sugar
- 200 g walnuts
- 3 tablespoon vegetable oil
- 500 ml water

For the glaze:

- A handful of chopped fresh herbs
- 1 egg
- 1 tablespoon water

Directions:

Mix all the flours along with the salt in a large bowl; add herbs and yeast and make a well in the middle. Mix together the sugar, water and oil and pour the mixture into the flour, mixing the ingredients until they form dough. Turn the dough onto a floured board, kneading it for 10 minutes. Then placing it into an oiled bowl, cover and leave it in a warm place until the size doubles. Preheat the oven to 200 degrees Celsius; knead the walnuts into the dough and divide it into eight portions; shape each portion into a roll and place it onto a greased baking pan. For the glaze, blench all the herbs in hot water for a few seconds and then place them in iced water. Mix together the water and egg and brush the rolls with this mixture; arrange the herbs on top and brush again. Bake for 12 – 15 minutes.

Chapter # 3: Rye Rounds

Makes: 8 – 10 servings

Cooking time: 15 minutes

Ingredients:

1. 4 cups shredded Cheddar cheese
2. ½ cup diced sweet onions
3. ½ cup mayonnaise
4. 1 loaf of cocktail rye bread
5. ½ cup, small pieces of boiled chicken

Directions:

Preheat the oven to broil. In a small mixing bowl, combine the cheese, mayonnaise, chicken and onion. Arrange the rye rounds on a baking sheet and spoon the mixture onto the bread. Broil until the mixture is hot making sure that the tops of the bread aren't burned.

Conclusion

Although wheat products rule the top shelves of most supermarkets, foods made from rye provide a greater bang for the consumer's buck. They are not only rich in nutrients and protect against deadly diseases but also are hearty in taste and satiating for the body. Once a food for the poor, it is not wrong to say that rye has established itself as one of the world's leading cereals when it comes to health-promoting features.

This book tells you everything, from rye's color to its storage techniques to its health benefits. In simple words, everything you need to know about rye has been given in the book; it is up to you now to follow the instructions and lead a happy life.

References

http://www.123rf.com/photo_7970890_ripe-rye-against-the-blue-sky.html?term=rye

http://www.123rf.com/photo_14902351_traditional-bread.html?term=rye

http://www.123rf.com/photo_29675919_cereals-in-sacks.html?term=rye%20storage

http://www.123rf.com/photo_13921125_gallstones.html?term=gallstones

http://www.fotolia.com/id/7367691

http://www.fotolia.com/id/39611032

http://www.fotolia.com/id/47136007

http://www.fotolia.com/id/49549245

Author Bio

Muhammad Usman is a distinguished medical graduate of Allama iqbal medical college (AIMC). He is a professional writer who has been in the field for more than 4 years. During this time he has produced 10,000+ articles, blogs and eBooks on various niches related to diseases, health, fitness, nutrition and well-being. He is a regular contributor to several journals related to medicine and surgery. He is the editor of several journals and newspapers.

Check out some of the other JD-Biz Publishing books

Gardening Series on Amazon

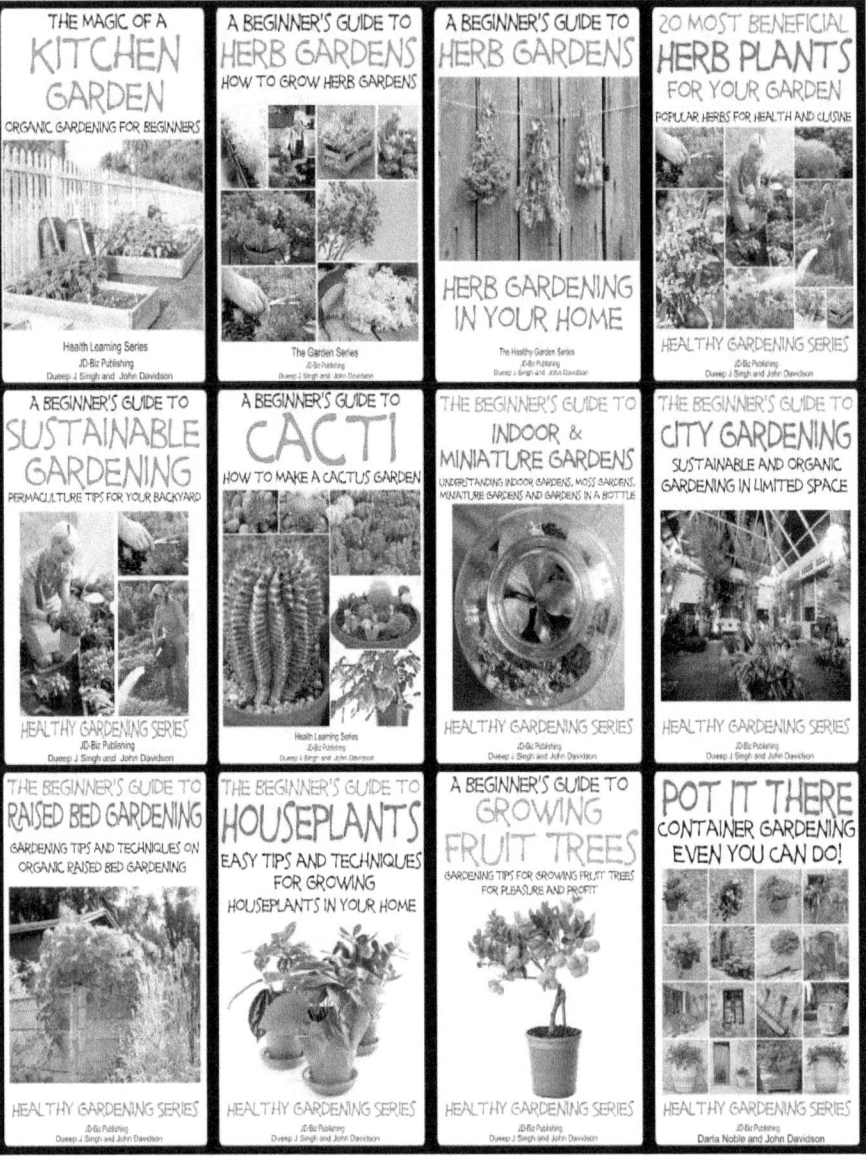

Health Learning Series

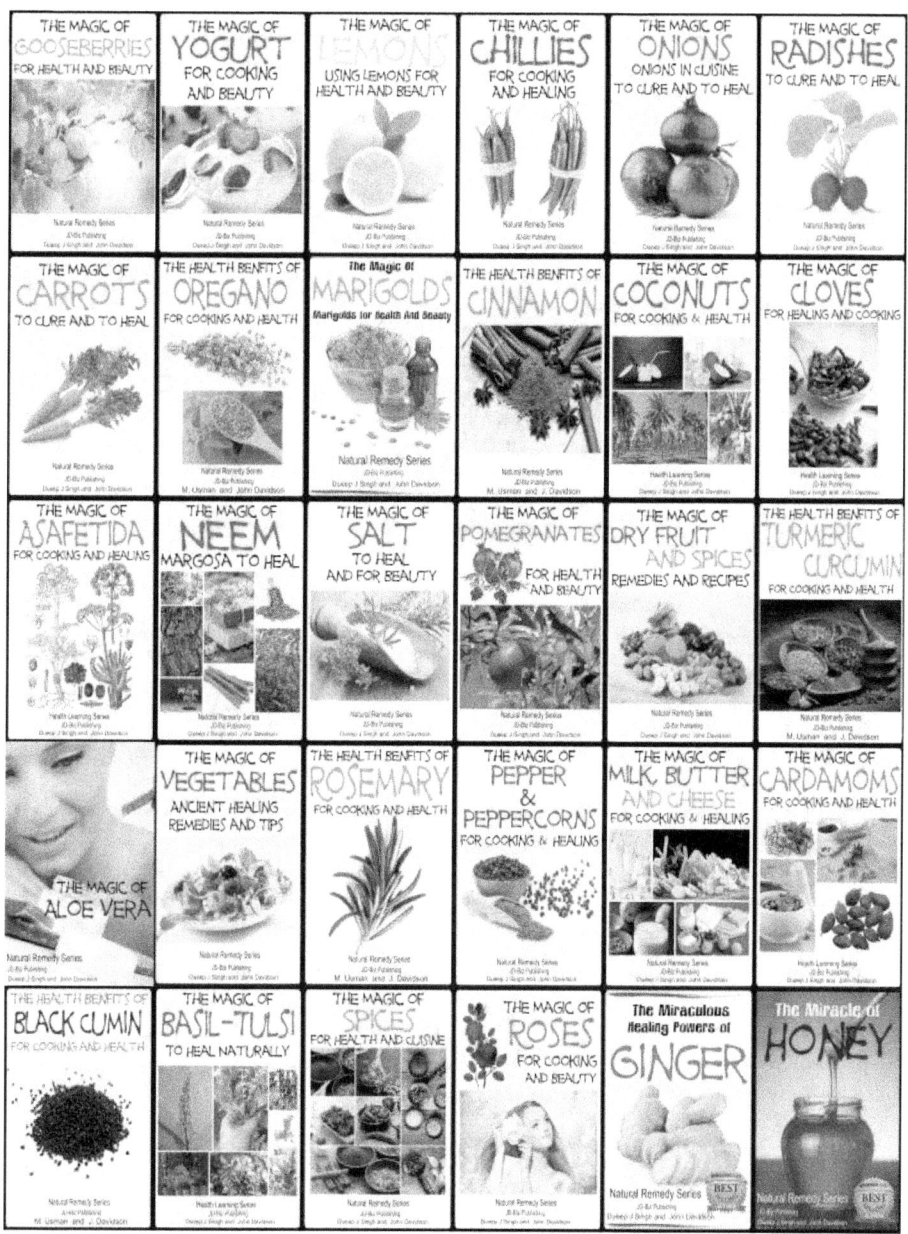

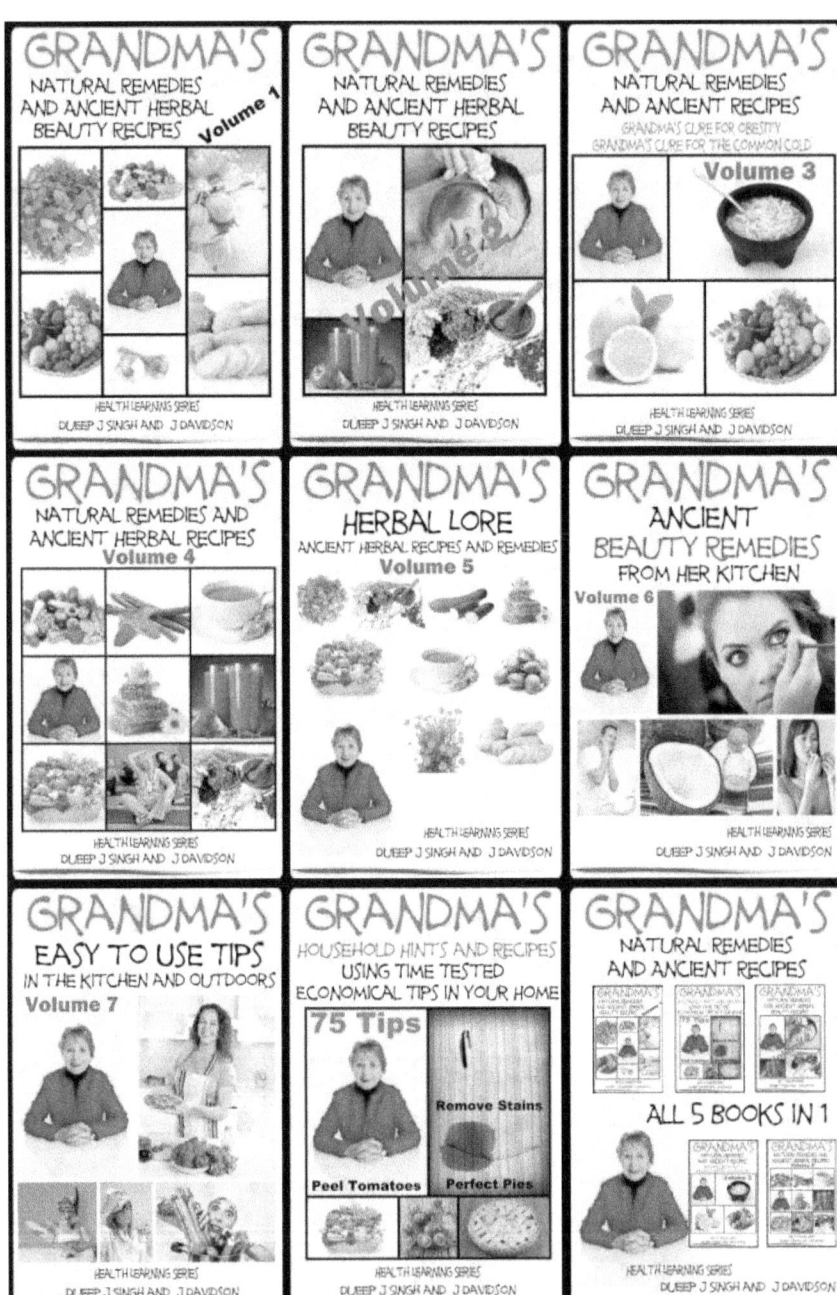

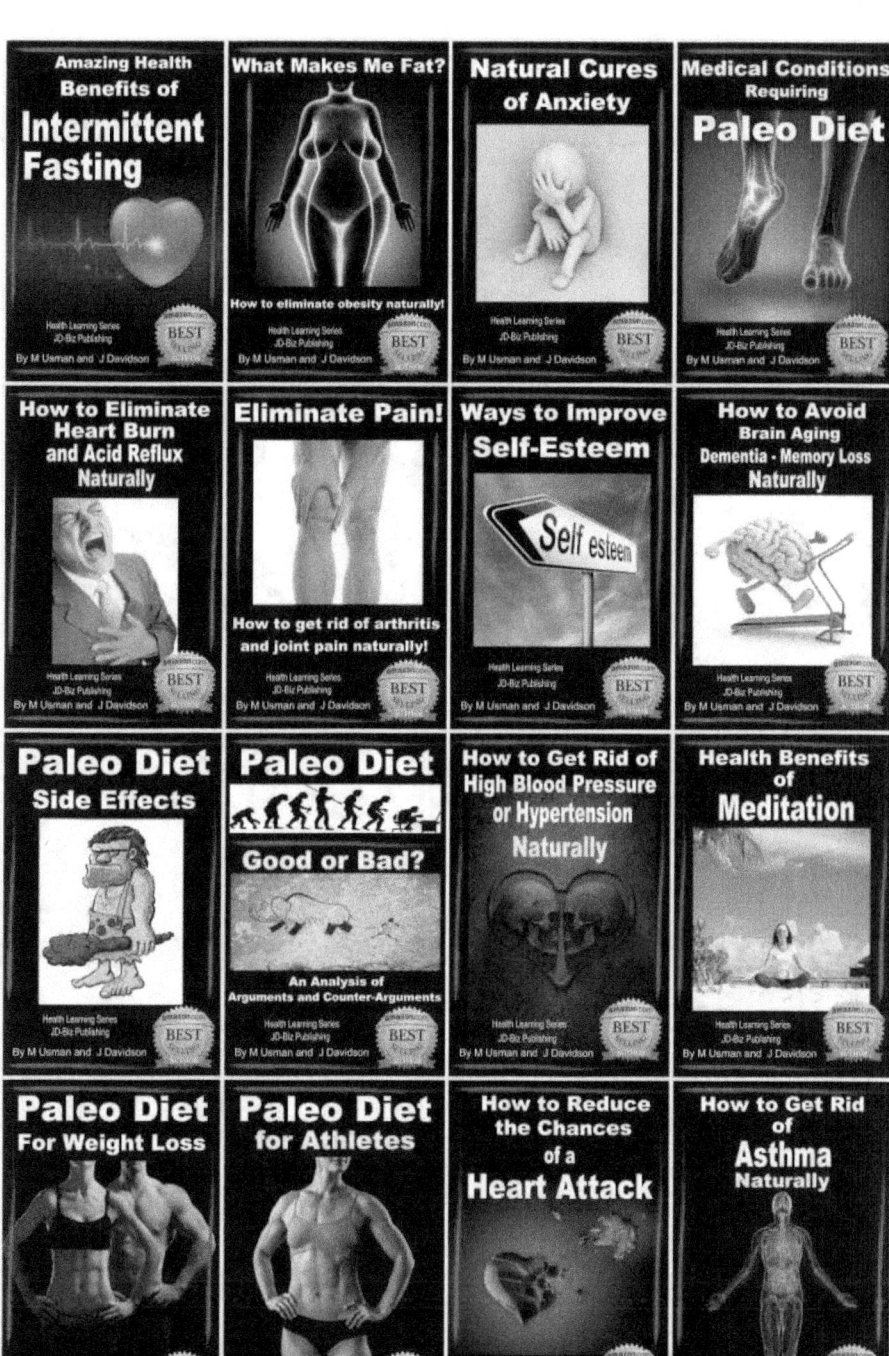

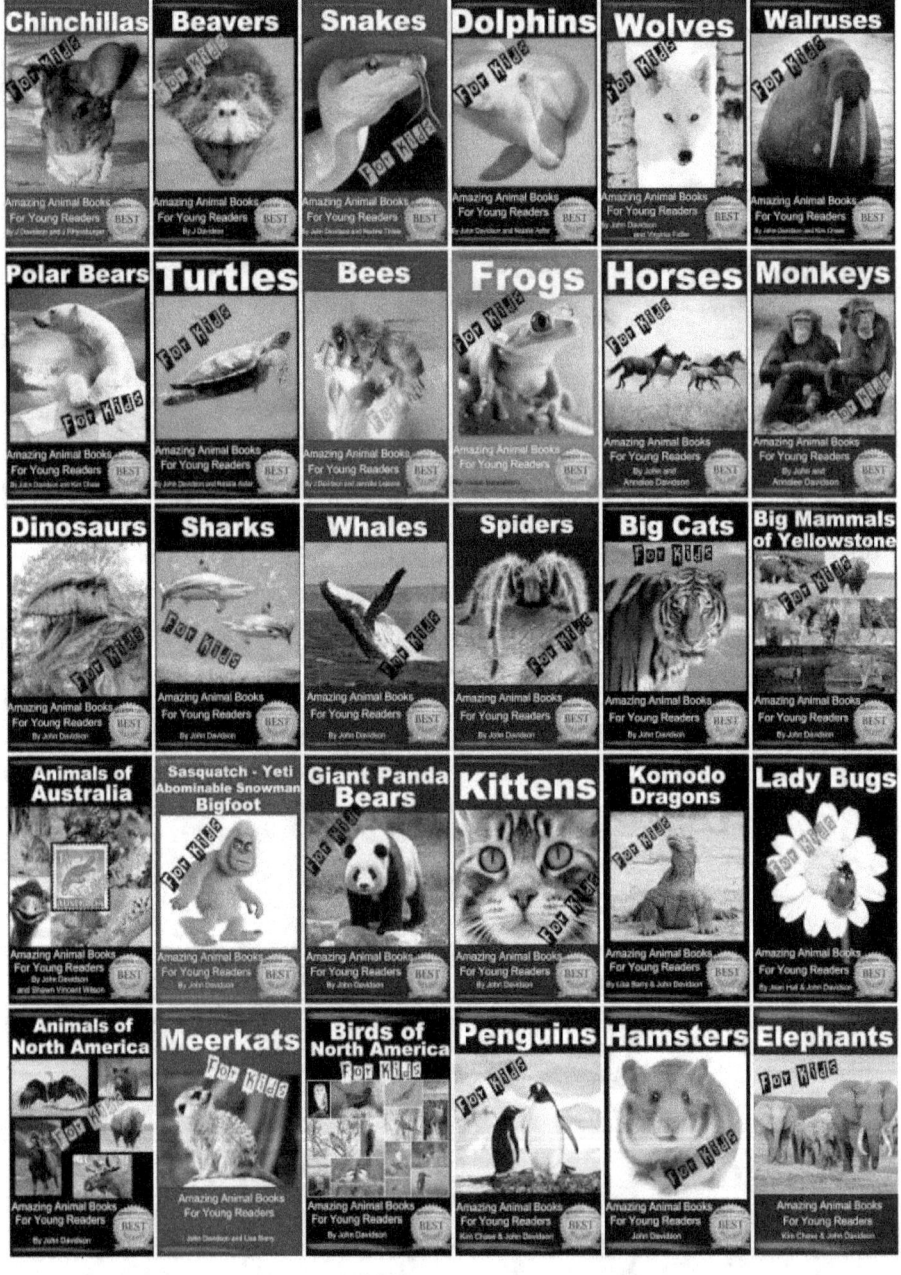

Learn To Draw Series

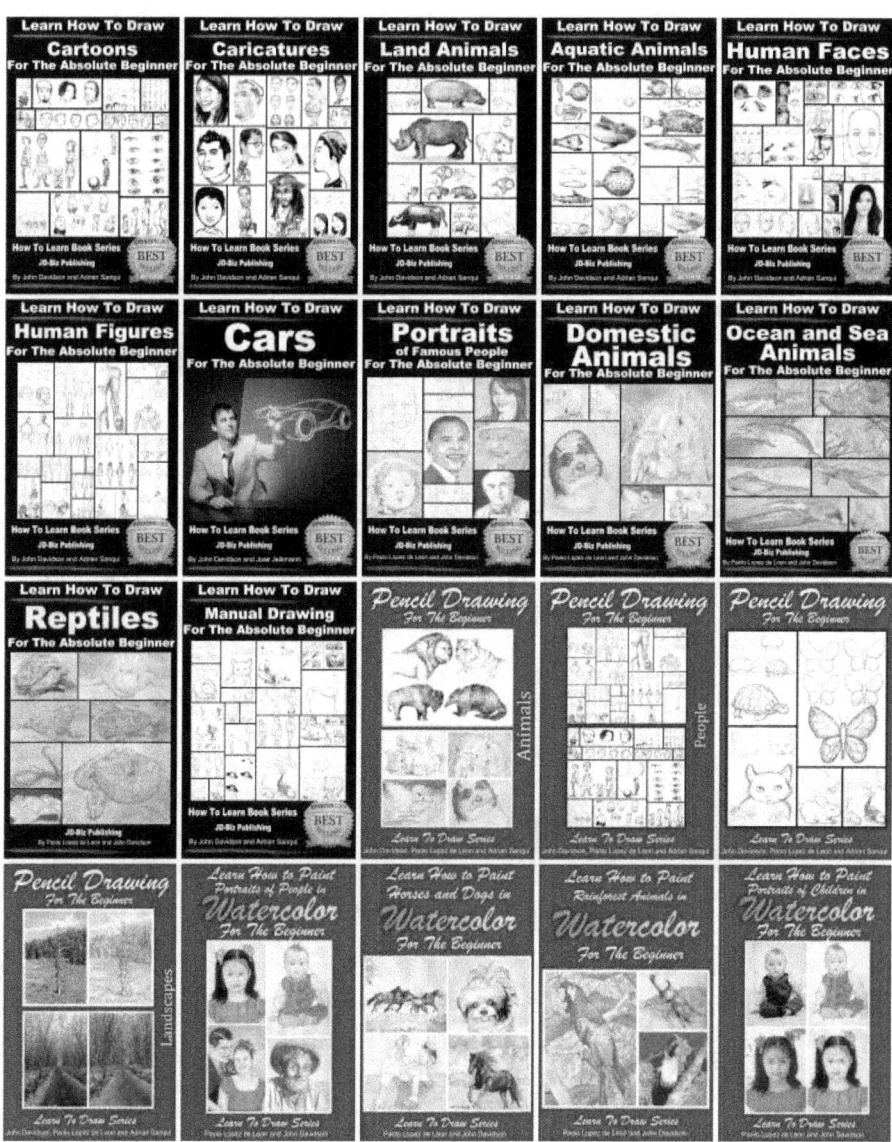

How to Build and Plan Books

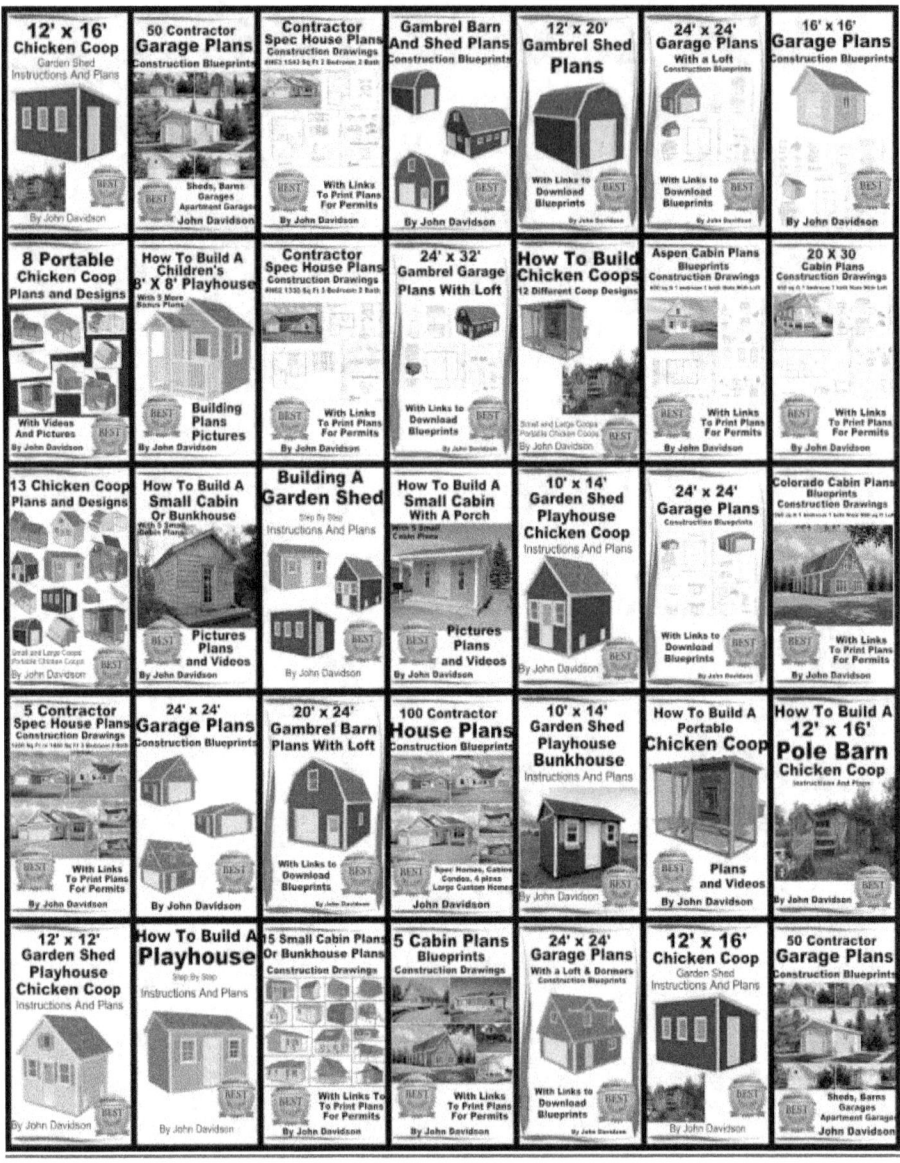

Entrepreneur Book Series

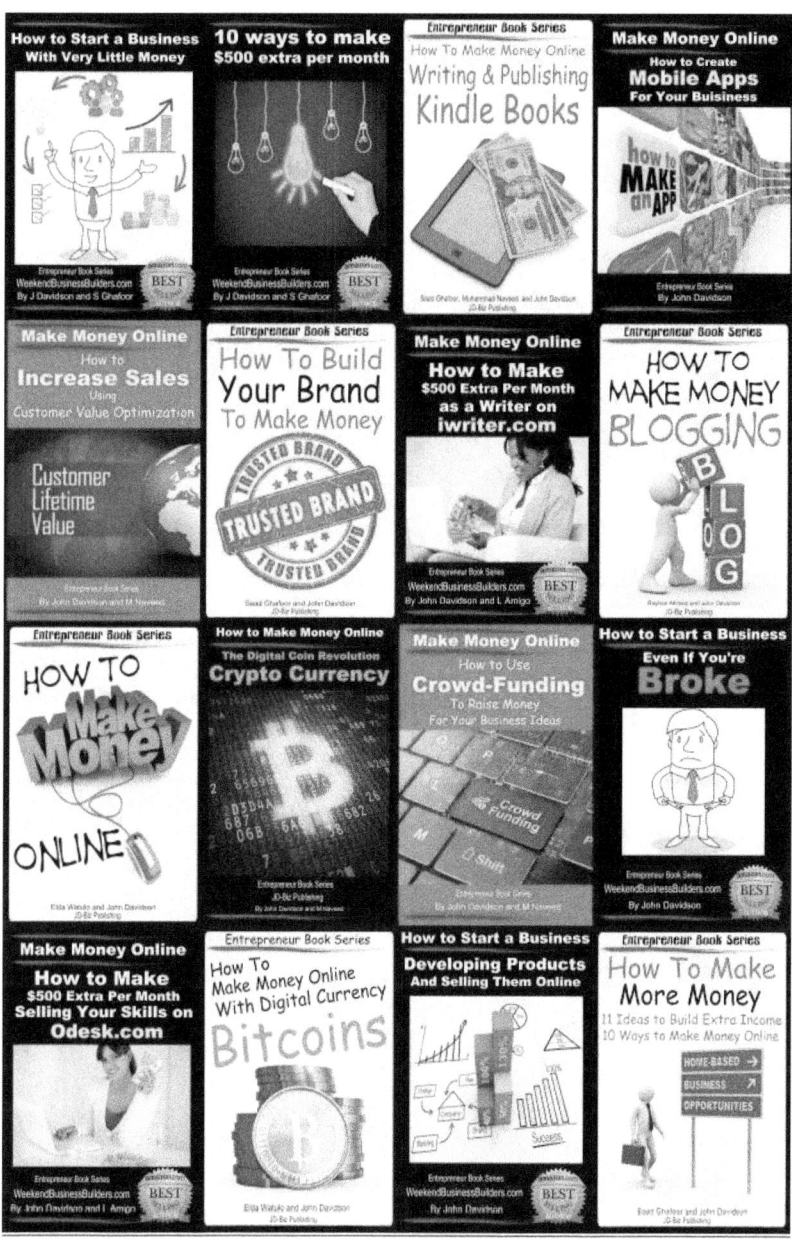

Our books are available at

1. Amazon.com

2. Barnes and Noble

3. Itunes

4. Kobo

5. Smashwords

6. Google Play Books

This book is published by

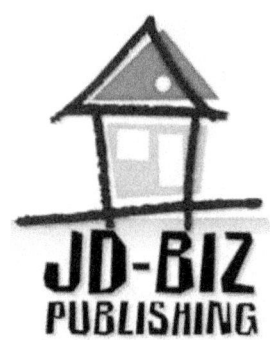

JD-Biz Corp

P O Box 374

Mendon, Utah 84325

http://www.jd-biz.com/

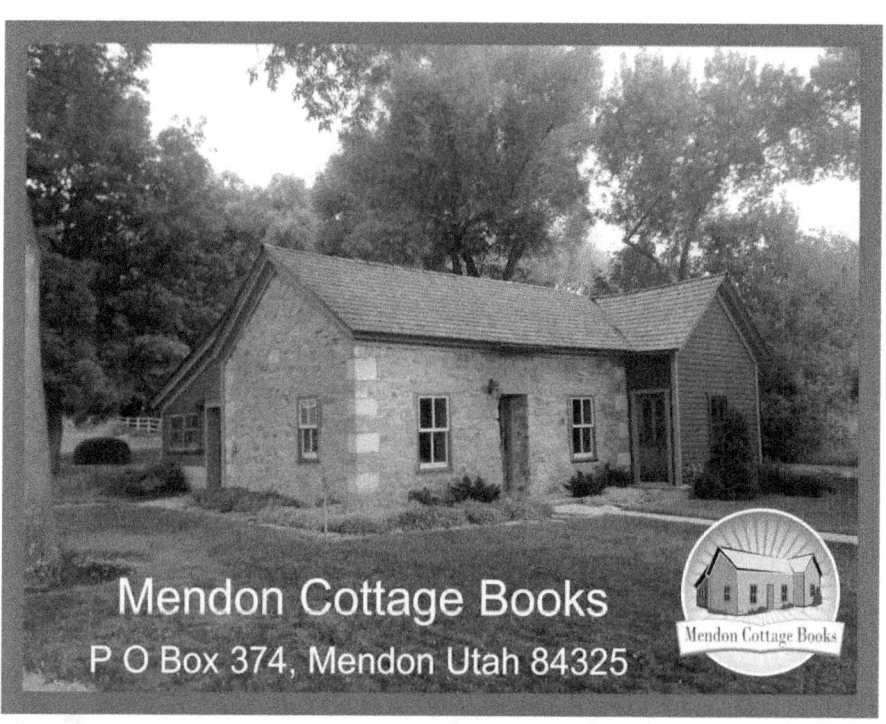

www.ingramcontent.com/pod-product-compliance
Lightning Source LLC
Chambersburg PA
CBHW061802280526
45787CB00003BA/1456

* 9 7 8 1 5 0 5 5 7 5 9 7 2 *